Neurology for MRCP PACES

HANI TS BENAMER

FRCP PhD

Consultant Neurologist

Honorary Clinical Senior Lecturer

The Royal Wolverhampton Hospitals NHS Trust

University Hospitals NHS Foundation Trust

University of Birmingham

Radcliffe Publishing
Oxford • New York

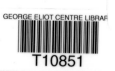

Radcliffe Publishing Ltd
18 Marcham Road
Abingdon
Oxon OX14 1AA
United Kingdom

www.radcliffe-oxford.com

Electronic catalogue and worldwide online ordering facility.

British Library Cataloguing in Publication Data

A catalogue record for this book is available from the British Library.

ISBN-13: 978 184619 397 2

The paper used for the text pages of this book
is FSC certified. FSC (The Forest Stewardship
Council) is an international network to promote
responsible management of the world's forests.

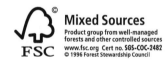

Mixed Sources
Product group from well-managed
forests and other controlled sources
www.fsc.org Cert no. SGS-COC-2482
© 1996 Forest Stewardship Council

Typeset by Pindar NZ, Auckland, New Zealand
Printed and bound by TJI Digital, Padstow, Cornwall, UK

Contents

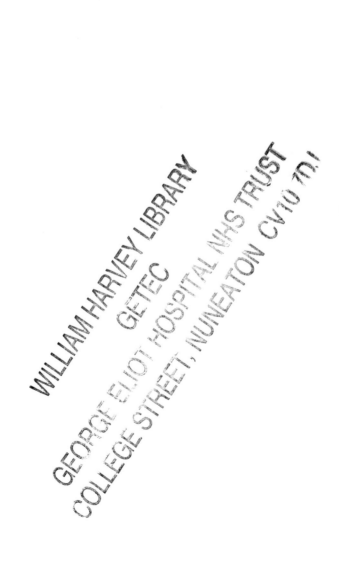

Preface

Neurology has the reputation of being difficult. Doctors who are sitting postgraduate exams fear, if not hate, the clinical neurology stations (PACES and traditional short cases), where they have to demonstrate their examination skills under very watchful eyes. Anxiety and panic intensify as the candidates have to present, in a very short time, an interpretation of the clinical findings, and discuss diagnosis, investigations and treatment possibilities. The main reason for all these emotions is the ease with which candidates could get lost in unnecessary details during the lengthy neurological examination. This book was put together to help to overcome this problem, to make life simple and to some extent demystify neurology.

The main aims of this book are as follows:

- to help candidates who are sitting clinical exams to arrange their thoughts in such a way as to enable them to respond quickly and adequately to the instructions that are commonly given in the neurology exam stations
- to polish their approach to the neurology examination
- to help to organise the clinical findings in a simple, short and presentable way
- to present simple and essential facts in an easy-to-remember format to help candidates to pass clinical neurology exam stations.

To help to achieve these aims, this book is divided into three major sections. Each section covers the areas of the human body usually examined in neurology, i.e. head and neck, upper limbs and lower limbs. Each section is organised according to the possible instructions that candidates may encounter in the exam. For example, the head and neck section has four sub-sections under the following headings: examine the cranial nerves; examine the eyes; examine the face; examine the speech. Within each sub-section there is a summary of the essential examination steps that have to be undertaken when responding to the instruction 'What should you do?', followed by the possible clinical findings. Under each finding there is a diagnosis followed by a brief discussion in question-and-answer format. All the way through, tips and pitfalls are listed.

This book assumes that the reader has some background knowledge in neurology and has practised the neurology examination. There are variations in how to examine neurological patients, and this book presents one of these variations that has been adapted by the author. To keep the content of the book simple and useful for the exam, there are inevitably some omissions. However, it is unlikely that you or your examiners (who are not usually neurologists) will be able to pick these up!

Finally, it is important to emphasise that no book can replace clinical experience. Therefore the best way to learn clinical medicine is, as you guessed, to see more patients!

Hani TS Benamer
January 2010

About the author

After graduating from Al-Fatah University, Tripoli, Libya in 1990, Hani came to the UK in 1991 to further his training in medicine. He obtained the MRCP in 1994 and trained in neurology at the Institute of Neurological Sciences in Glasgow. He obtained a PhD and CCST (Certificate of Completion of Specialist Training) in neurology in 2000, and was appointed a consultant neurologist in Wolverhampton and Birmingham the same year. He has been the lead neurologist at New Cross Hospital in Wolverhampton since 2006.

Hani has an interest in medical education, and obtained a post-graduate certificate in the field from Keele University in 2007. He has published more than 30 papers, and is currently one of the editors of the *Libyan Journal of Medicine*. He was also an examiner for the MRCP Diploma from 2005 to 2009.

Acknowledgements

I would like to thank all of the following colleagues, who kindly gave constructive comments on the manuscript of this book (or parts of it): Dr Seema Kalra, Dr John Winer, Dr Domnick D'Costa, Dr Paramjeet Deol and Dr Nicholas Davies.

I am also indebted to all of my teachers who taught me how to be a clinical neurologist. They are too many to mention.

List of abbreviations

CT	Computerised tomography
CTA	Computerised tomographic angiography
CTV	Computerised tomographic venogram
EMG	Electromyography
ESR	Erythrocyte sedimentation rate
LMN	Lower motor neurone
MRA	Magnetic resonance angiography
MRI	Magnetic resonance imaging
MRV	Magnetic resonance venogram
NCS	Nerve conduction study
PACES	Practical Assessment of Clinical Examination Skills
UMN	Upper motor neurone

To my wife and best friend
Hiba

SECTION I

Examination of the head and neck

INSTRUCTION A

Examine the cranial nerves

Instruction A: Examine the cranial nerves
What should you do?
First do the essential. This should include the following:

Look at the face
- Reduced forehead wrinkles (nerve VII).
- Ptosis (nerve III).
- Wasting of the temporalis muscles (nerve V).
- Absence of the nasolabial folds (nerve VII).

Ask the patient to
- Raise the eyebrows (nerve VII).
- Shut the eyes tightly. You should try to force them open (nerve VII).
- Blow out the cheeks (nerve VII).
- Show the teeth or smile (nerve VII).

Examine the eyes
- Be sure that the patient can see by checking their visual acuity using a (pocket) Snellen chart, with glasses. Alternatively, if a Snellen chart is not available, a newspaper or something similar could be used instead (nerve II).
- Look at the size of the pupils and their reaction to light, direct and indirect responses (nerves II/III).
- Do the eye movements and ask if there is double vision (nerves III, IV and VI).
- Examine the fundi, mainly looking at the optic discs (nerve II).

Examine the face
- Test pinprick sensation in the upper, middle and lower part of the face (the three divisions of nerve V).
- Palpate the masseter and temporalis muscles by asking the patient to clench the teeth (nerve V).

Examine the mouth
- Ask the patient to open the jaw against your hand (nerve V).
- Inspect the tongue inside the floor of the mouth (nerve XII).
- Ask the patient to protrude the tongue (nerve XII).
- Ask the patient to move the tongue from side to side, and look for any slowness (nerve XII).
- Ask the patient to say 'Ah', and assess the movement of the soft palate and the uvula (nerve X).

Examine the neck and the shoulders
- Ask the patient to twist the head to one direction against your hand. Palpate the opposite sternomastoid (nerve XI).
- Ask the patient to shrug the shoulders against resistance (nerve XI).

Tips
- If you finish the above examination and find no abnormalities, examine the visual field by confrontation. Using a white hat pin, sit at the same level as the patient, about 1 metre away, compare your field to the patient and test the four quadrants. A red pin is used to test for central scotoma (rarely necessary in routine neurology practice or exam!).
- If abnormal signs are still not detected, you have most probably missed the signs, or you are unlucky enough to have a normal patient!
- If you found abnormalities in the pupil size, test the reaction of the pupils to convergence by asking the patient to look straight ahead and then at the tip of their nose.
- If you find evidence of Vth nerve impairment, do the corneal reflex. Remember to stimulate the cornea, not the sclera.
- If there is VIIth nerve palsy, test for evidence of sensori-neural deafness (nerve VIII), or at least ask if the patient has any hearing difficulties.

- Always think as you are examining the patient. It is a good idea to have a summary of the findings in your head before reporting to the examiner.

FINDINGS

Finding One

Unilateral, partial or complete ptosis with eye deviating laterally (down and out) with or without pupillary dilatation. Impaired response to light and accommodation.

Diagnosis
- (Right or left) (complete or partial) IIIrd nerve palsy.

Tips
- Make sure that it is an isolated IIIrd nerve palsy and that there is no evidence of nerve V (especially V1 and V2 sensory impairments) and VIth nerve involvement.
- It can be difficult to ascertain whether there is IVth nerve involvement. Nerve IV supplies the superior oblique, which suppresses the adducted eye. With a IIIrd nerve palsy the patient would not be able to adduct the affected eye, so when they are asked to move the eye downward the eye will rotate inward if nerve IV is intact.
- IIIrd nerve palsy causes ptosis, as it innervates the levator palpebrae muscle.
- IIIrd nerve palsy could cause a fixed dilated pupil with paralysis of accommodation, as it carries the parasympathetic fibre to the pupil.

Discussion
Q: What are the causes of IIIrd nerve palsy?
- Ischaemic (microvascular) IIIrd nerve palsy. Usually painless with pupillary sparing in patients with diabetes and/or hypertension.
- Surgical causes such as posterior communicating artery aneurysm (painful) or brainstem tumour.
- Multiple sclerosis and migraine rarely cause an isolated IIIrd nerve palsy.
- IIIrd nerve palsy could be due to uncal herniation (an

important sign to recognise in clinical practice, but not in the exam!).

- If there is involvement of the V (V1 and V2) and VI, a lesion in the superior orbital fissure or cavernous sinus should be considered (metastasis, sphenoid wing meningioma, nasopharyngeal carcinoma, carotid siphon aneurysm or cavernous sinus thrombosis).
- Basal meningeal lesion as a result of infection (tuberculosis or fungal), carcinomatous, neurosarcoid or direct spread from nasopharyngeal tumour.

Q: How would you investigate?
- Check for diabetes.
- Brain MRI and/or MRA (CTA could be used instead of MRA).
- Cerebrospinal fluid analysis if there is a possibility of a basal meningeal lesion.

Q: What is the treatment?
- Spontaneous recovery in patients with ischaemic IIIrd nerve palsy, usually within 3 months.
- Treat the underlying cause, which may involve surgery.

Finding Two

Horizontally separated double vision on looking to the right/left with limitation of abduction of right/left eye. The outer image disappears when the right/left eye is covered.

Diagnosis
- (Right or left) VIth nerve palsy.

Tips
- The outer image is always the false one. It disappears when the affected eye is covered.
- Check the fundi for papilloedema.

Discussion
Q: What are the causes of VIth nerve palsy?
- Ischaemic (microvascular) VIth nerve palsy (especially in patients with diabetes and hypertension).
- False localising sign due to increased intracranial pressure (*see* page 17).
- Brainstem lesions such as tumour or demyelination (multiple sclerosis).
- If there is involvement of other cranial nerves, such as nerves III, IV and V, consider superior orbital fissure, cavernous sinus or basal meningeal lesion (*see* page 11).

Q: How would you investigate?
- Brain MRI.

Q: What is the treatment?
- Spontaneous recovery occurs in ischaemic VIth nerve palsy, usually within 3 months.
- Treat the underlying cause.
- Prism to correct the double vision.

Finding Three

(a) Visual field assessment showed evidence of impairment of both temporal fields.
(b) Visual field assessment showed evidence of impairment of the temporal field on one side and the nasal field on the other side.

Diagnosis
- (a) Bitemporal hemianopia as a result of a lesion in the optic chiasma.
- (b) Homonymous hemianopia as a result of an optic tract lesion.

Tips
- Assessment of the visual field by confrontation can be crude. Therefore it is less likely that you will get patients with superior quadrantanopia (temporal lobe lesion) or inferior quadrantanopia (parietal lobe lesion).
- Homonymous hemianopia is due to a lesion behind the optic chiasma. The visual field defect in this case is on the contralateral side of the lesion (e.g. a lesion in the *right* posterior optic tract causes *left* homonymous hemianopia).

Discussion
Q: What are the causes of the visual field defect?
- (a) Bitemporal hemianopia is usually caused by pituitary tumour. Other causes include craniopharyngioma, meningioma and large internal carotid artery aneurysm.
- (b) Homonymous hemianopia is usually caused by cerebrovascular disease such as occipital infarction or haemorrhage. Other causes include tumours.

Q: How would you investigate?
- Brain MRI.
- Hormonal assessment in the case of a pituitary tumour.

- Formal assessment of the visual field by Goldmann perimetry or the Humphrey technique.

Q: What is the treatment?
- Treat the underlying cause. Urgent surgery for pituitary tumour may be needed to save the vision.

Finding Four

Pale optic disc (with sharp margins).

Diagnosis
- Optic atrophy.

Tips
- Check for relative afferent pupillary defect by the light swing test (swing the light from one pupil to the other every one or two seconds). Normal pupils constrict every time they are exposed to light. In relative afferent pupillary defect, the pupil dilates when exposed to light.
- Testing for central scotoma using the red pin will only confirm the obvious, and is probably not necessary.

Discussion
Q: What are the causes of optic atrophy?
- Multiple sclerosis in young patients.
- Ischaemic optic neuropathy in elderly patients.
- Other causes include optic nerve compression, Leber's hereditary optic neuropathy, toxins (tobacco and methyl alcohol) and nutritional deficiencies (vitamin B_1 and vitamin B_{12}).
- If the atrophy is associated with ill defined disc margins, consider secondary optic atrophy due to long-standing papilloedema.

Q: How would you investigate?
- Brain MRI.

Q: What is the treatment?
- Treat the underlying cause if possible.

Finding Five

Absent venous pulsation and blurring of optic disc margin with or without haemorrhages or exudates.

Diagnosis
- Optic disc swelling (bilateral papilloedema).

Tips
- Papilloedema is an optic disc swelling due to raised intracranial pressure. Therefore 'optic disc swelling' is the more correct term.
- Check for any evidence of VIth nerve palsy.

Discussion
Q: What are the causes of papilloedema?
- Increased intracranial pressure due to brain tumours, cerebrovenous sinus thrombosis and cerebral abscess.
- In a young obese female patient the likely diagnosis is idiopathic (benign) intracranial hypertension.
- Other rare causes include malignant hypertension, cavernous sinus thrombosis and Guillain–Barré syndrome.

Q: What are the other causes of optic disc swelling?
- Papillitis: acute inflammation of the optic nerve, usually due to multiple sclerosis.

Q: How could you differentiate between papillitis and papilloedema?
- Papillitis causes visual loss, whereas visual acuity is normal (until a very late stage) in papilloedema.
- Papillitis causes central scotoma, whereas papilloedema causes constriction of the peripheral visual fields.
- Papillitis causes retro-orbital pain, whereas patients with papilloedema may experience generalised headache.

- Papillitis causes afferent pupillary defect (*see* page 16), whereas in papilloedema the pupils are normal.

Q: How would you investigate?
- Brain CT/MRI and MRV (CTV could be used instead of MRV).
- Lumbar puncture to measure the pressure in idiopathic (benign) intracranial hypertension.

Q: What is the treatment?
- Treatment of the underlying tumour or abscess.
- Administration of diuretics such as acetazolamide and weight loss in idiopathic intracranial hypertension.
- Consider anticoagulation in cerebrovenous sinus thrombosis.
- Steroids may be given to patients with papillitis.

Finding Six

Right/left facial weakness involving the whole side of the face. Difficulty with raising the right/left eyebrow, inability to shut the right/left eye fully. Bell's phenomenon, difficulty with cheek blowing, obliteration of the right/left nasolabial fold and droopy mouth.

Diagnosis
- (Right or left) LMN VIIth nerve palsy.

Tips
- Bell's phenomenon is the turning of the eye upward when the patient is asked to shut the eyes.
- The mouth deviates to the normal side in VIIth nerve palsy, leading to a droopy mouth on the side of the lesion.
- Hyperacusis could be a feature of VIIth nerve palsy.
- Check for any vesicles around the external auditory meatus.
- Check for any enlargement of the parotid gland.
- Check for any evidence of surgical scars.
- Make sure that nerves V, VI and VIII are intact.
- If you find that you get confused by the Rinne's and Weber's test, ask whether the patient has any hearing impairment, or rub your thumb and index finger near the patient's ear while blocking the other ear.
- Bilateral LMN lesion of nerve VII could be difficult to detect due to absence of asymmetry. If you find bilateral VIIth nerve palsy, ask whether you could examine the upper and lower limbs, especially for weakness and absent reflexes.
- Myasthenia and muscle disease such as fascio-scapulo-humeral dystrophy could lead to bilateral facial weakness which mimics bilateral facial palsy.

Discussion
Q: What are the causes of LMN VIIth nerve palsy?
- Bell's palsy.

19

- Ramsey–Hunt syndrome due to herpes zoster infection.
- Cerebello-pontine angle lesion such as acoustic neuroma (if nerves V and/or VIII are affected).
- Head injuries involving the petrous bone.
- Middle ear infection.
- Parotid tumour.
- Parotid gland or ear surgery.
- Pontine lesion such as tumour if nerves V and/or VI are involved.
- Rarely caused by multiple sclerosis and neurosarcoid.
- If it is bilateral, consider Guillain–Barré syndrome, neurosarcoid and Lyme disease.

Q: How would you investigate?
- This depends on the possible cause. No investigation is needed in Bell's palsy. Brain MRI for central lesion. NCS/EMG if Guillain–Barré syndrome is suspected.

Q: What is the treatment?
- Spontaneous full recovery occurs in more than 80% of patients with Bell's palsy. The role of steroids and acyclovir is still controversial. However, they are commonly used, especially if the patient is seen within 72 hours of the onset of the palsy.
- Treat the underlying cause.

Finding Seven

(a) Wasted and atrophic tongue with fasciculation.
(b) Small, slow-moving spastic tongue.
(c) Slow-moving wasted and atrophic tongue with fasciculation.

Diagnosis
- (a) Bulbar palsy (bilateral lower motor lesion of nerve XII).
- (b) Pseudobulbar palsy (bilateral upper motor lesion of nerve XII).
- (c) Mixture of both bulbar and pseudobulbar palsy.

Tips
- Check the jaw reflex. A brisk reflex is an indicator of pseudobulbar palsy.
- Ask whether you could examine the patient's speech (nasal quality in bulbar palsy and spastic slurring dysarthria in pseudobulbar palsy).
- Swallowing is usually impaired in both bulbar and pseudobulbar palsy.
- Emotional lability is a feature of pseudobulbar palsy.
- Look for evidence of bilateral LMN lesion of nerve X (poor movement of the soft palate).

Discussion
Q: What are the causes of bulbar palsy?
- Motor neurone disease.
- Syringobulbia.
- Skull base lesion which is usually due to cancer (nerve VII could also be involved).
- Brainstem tumour.

Q: What are the causes of pseudobulbar palsy?
- Extensive cerebrovascular disease causing bilateral ischaemia.

- Motor neurone disease.

Q: What are the causes of the mixture of bulbar and pseudobulbar palsy?
- Motor neurone disease.

Q: How would you investigate?
According to the likely cause:
- NCS/EMG.
- Brain MRI.
- Cerebrospinal fluid analysis.

Q: What is the treatment?
- Riluzole in motor neurone disease.
- Treatment of the underlying cause if possible.

Finding Eight

Unilateral wasting and fasciculation of the tongue. Deviation of the tongue to one side.

Diagnosis
- Unilateral LMN lesion of nerve XII.

Tips
- The tongue deviates *towards* the side of the lesion.
- Check nerves IX and X, as they may be affected.

Discussion
Q: What are the causes of XIIth nerve palsy?
- Basal meningitis due to cancer, lymphoma, tuberculosis or sarcoidosis.
- Syringobulbia.
- Foramen magnum tumour.
- Nasopharyngeal tumour.

Q: How would you investigate?
- Brain and/or cervical MRI.
- Cerebrospinal fluid analysis.

Q: What is the treatment?
- Treat the underlying cause.

Finding Nine

Poor movement of the soft palate with deviation of the uvula. Weakness in twisting the head and shrugging the shoulders.

Diagnosis
- Right/left Xth and XIth nerve palsy (jugular foramen syndrome).

Tips
- The uvula deviates *away* from the side of the lesion. However, the deviation of midline soft palate could be a better indicator than the uvula.
- Nerve IX is usually involved, but it is mainly a sensory nerve. Therefore it is not assessed formally in the exam.
- The sternomastoid muscle turns the head in the *opposite* direction (e.g. weakness in twisting the head to the *right* is due to weakness of the *left* sternomastid).
- Check the tongue, as a lesion in the jugular foramen could spread to involve nerve XII.

Discussion
Q: What are the causes of jugular foramen syndrome?
- Tumours such as neurofibroma, meningioma and glomus jugulare tumour.
- Carcinomatous infiltration.
- Neurosarcoid.
- Infection spreading from middle ear disease.

Q: How would you investigate?
- Brain MRI.
- Cerebrospinal fluid analysis.

Q: What is the treatment?
- Treatment of the underlying cause, which could involve surgery.

INSTRUCTION B

Examine the eyes

Instruction B: Examine the eyes
What should you do?

- Look for any evidence of ptosis.
- Be sure that the patient can see by checking their visual acuity using a (pocket) Snellen chart, with glasses. If a Snellen chart is not available, a newspaper or something similar could be used instead.
- Look at the size of the pupils and their reaction to light (direct and indirect responses).
- Do the eye movements and ask whether there is double vision.
- Look specifically for nystagmus.
- If you find no abnormalities, look at the fundi and do the visual fields.

Tips

- If you are allowed to talk to the patient, ask them the following questions: 'Do you see normally out of both eyes? Do you have double vision? Is it horizontally or vertically separated? And in what direction does it get worse?'
- Always remember myasthenia as a possible diagnosis if you are asked to examine the eyes. Try to demonstrate fatigability.
- You are unlikely to be given a case where nystagmus is the only finding. You are more likely to find nystagmus as part of cerebellar syndrome (*see* page 111). Make sure that you are not missing internuclear ophthalmoplegia.
- The majority of findings that you may encounter, if you are asked to examine the eyes, are covered under Instruction A: Examine the cranial nerves (*see* pages 11, 13, 14, 16 and 17).

FINDINGS

Finding One

Bilateral, variable, fatigable and asymmetrical ptosis with evidence of a varying degree of diplopia and ophthalmoplegia.

Diagnosis
- Myasthenia gravis.

Tips
- Look for fatigability by asking the patient to keep looking upward for a minute. The ptosis usually gets worse.
- Look for any evidence of facial weakness.
- Ask whether you could examine the patient's speech.
- Ask whether the patient has any problems with swallowing.
- Look for any evidence of weakness of the neck muscles (mainly extensors) by asking the patient to push their head backward against your hand (the patient may be supporting the head by pushing the chin upward).
- Ask whether you could examine the upper and lower limbs for any evidence of weakness.

Discussion
Q: How would you confirm the diagnosis?
- Edrophonium (Tensilon) test or ice pack test.
- Check the acetylcholine-receptor antibodies (positive in more than 90% in generalised myasthenia and 50% in ocular myasthenia).
- EMG and single-fibre EMG.

Q: What other investigations would you perform?
- CT or MRI of the chest, looking for any evidence of thymoma.

Q: What is the treatment?
- Monitor and support the respiratory function if necessary.

The patient may require regular measurement of forced vital capacity. Patients in acute myasthenic crisis require intubation and ventilation.

- Thymectomy if there is evidence of thymoma. Thymectomy is also indicated in young patients with generalised myasthenia.
- Pyridostigmine (anticholinesterase) as symptomatic treatment.
- Immunosuppression, including oral prednisolone and/or azathioprine.
- Intravenous immunoglobulin and plasmapheresis could be used in severe cases and during acute myasthenic crisis.

Finding Two

Unilateral incomplete ptosis with no evidence of abnormal eye movement. Pupil is small and reacts to light and accommodation.

Diagnosis
- Right/left-sided Horner's syndrome.

Tips
- The patient may show evidence of enophthalmos and lack of sweating on the side of the lesion.
- Horner's syndrome is due to a lesion in the sympathetic pathway. The lesion could occur at the hypothalamus, medulla, cervical cord or sympathetic chain.
- Look for any evidence of wasting of the small muscles of the hand.
- Look for any evidence of a surgical scar on the neck.
- Look for any evidence of neck trauma.
- Does the patient have any evidence of lower cranial nerve abnormalities?
- Ask the examiners whether the patient experienced pain at the onset of the symptoms.

Discussion
Q: What are the causes of Horner's syndrome?
- Isolated painless Horner's syndrome could be idiopathic.
- Pancoast's syndrome as a result of apical lung malignancy.
- Trauma or surgery, such as thyroid surgery.
- Thoracic outlet syndrome.
- Painful Horner's syndrome could be associated with migraine and carotid artery dissection. Other causes include syringomyelia, nasopharyngeal cancer and lateral medullary syndrome.

Q: How would you investigate?

- This depends on the possible causes. The patient usually requires MRI of the brain and cervical spine together with a chest X-ray.

Q: What is the treatment?

- Treat the underlying cause if possible.

Finding Three

When the patient looks to the right/left, there is ataxic nystagmus in the abducted eye and failure to adduct the other eye. The patient has internuclear ophthalmoplegia.

Diagnosis
- Multiple sclerosis.

Tips
- When you cover the abducted eye, the adduction in the other eye is normal.
- Ask whether you could look for any evidence of multiple sclerosis, such as spastic legs, ataxia or optic atrophy.

Discussion
Q: Where is the lesion?
- In the medial longitudinal fasciculus which connects the nerve III nucleus on one side with the nerve VI nucleus on the other side.

Q: What are the other causes of internuclear ophthalmoplegia?
- Cerebrovascular disease.

Q: How would you investigate this patient?
- MRI of the brain.
- Cerebrospinal fluid analysis looking for oligoclonal bands.

INSTRUCTION C

Examine the face

Instruction C: Examine the face
What should you do?

- You should follow the same steps as in the examination of cranial nerves (*see* page 5).
- Modify the steps according to your finding, i.e if you find ptosis, concentrate on the eyes and work through the differential diagnosis of ptosis.

Tips

- You are unlikely to be asked to examine the face of a patient with Parkinson's disease. You are more likely to encounter a case of Parkinson's disease when you are asked to examine the gait or the upper limbs. If this is the case, you need to demonstrate all of the parkinsonian features (*see* page 113).

FINDINGS

Finding One

Bilateral and symmetrical ptosis with frontal baldness, wasting of temporalis muscles and bilateral facial weakness. Evidence of myotonia. There may be some evidence of distal wasting of the arms and legs.

Diagnosis
- Myotonic dystrophy.

Tips
- Myotonia could be demonstrated by asking the patient to make a tight fist and release it. There will be a delay in relaxing the hand.
- Try to demonstrate percussion myotonia by striking the thenar eminence with a tendon hammer. It will take a long time for the dimple to return to normal.
- Look for any evidence of cataract surgery.
- Reflexes are absent.
- You may be instructed to examine the upper or lower limbs. Once you have recognised myotonia and distal weakness, the diagnosis should then be easy.

Discussion
Q: What are the other features of myotonic dystrophy?
- Cardiac conduction defects.
- Diabetes.
- Testicular atrophy.
- Impairment of intellectual function.

Q: What is the mode of inheritance?
- Autosomal dominant.

Q: How would you confirm the diagnosis?
- Send for DNA analysis, looking for the trinucleotide repeat expansion (CTG or CCTG).
- EMG.

Q: How would you manage this patient?
- Cardiac monitoring with regular ECG.
- Regular checking of blood sugar levels.
- Genetic counselling.

INSTRUCTION D

Examine the speech

Instruction D: Examine the speech
What should you do?

In examination of speech, the two most important aspects are comprehension (understanding) and fluency (spontaneous speech). These should be examined together by:

Asking questions
- 'What is your address?'
- 'What do you do for a living?'
- 'What did you have for breakfast?'
- Ask the patient to describe their job or what they have eaten in some detail, to help you to assess the speech.

Giving commands. Start with simple commands and increase the complexity as appropriate.
- 'Close your eyes.'
- 'Show me your right hand.'
- 'Close your right eye and touch your left ear with your right hand.'

Assessing repetition
- Ask the patient to repeat a simple word, such as 'pen' or 'watch.'
- Try a full sentence, such as 'It is very cold today.'
- Try a complicated phrase, such as 'No ifs, ands or buts.'

Tips
- The cortical area of speech is in the dominant hemisphere (the left hemisphere in right-handed people and in 60–70% of left-handed people).
- The speech has four components, namely comprehension of the language, production of language, articulation of the speech and phonation (sound and volume).
- Dysphasia is the impairment of comprehension or production of language. Dysarthria is the impairment of articulation. Dysphonia is the impairment of phonation.

- The anatomy of speech includes the superior temporal gyrus (Wernicke's area), inferior frontal gyrus (Broca's area), arcuate fasciculus (perisylvian region), which connects the superior temporal gyrus with the inferior frontal gyrus, corticobulbar pathway, cerebellum, basal ganglia, and cranial nerves V, VII, X and XII.
- You are unlikely to be asked to assess speech in a patient with dysarthria or dysphonia. You may encounter dysarthria as part of cerebellar syndrome (*see* page 111) or bulbar and pseudobulbar palsy (*see* page 21).

FINDINGS

Finding One

(a) Patient's comprehension is impaired. However, the speech is very fluent but does not make any sense (unintelligible). Repetition is impaired.
(b) Patient's comprehension is preserved but the speech is not fluent. Repetition is impaired.

Diagnosis
- (a) Receptive (sensory, fluent, Wernicke's, posterior) aphasia (dysphasia).
- (b) Expressive (motor, non-fluent, Broca's, anterior) aphasia (dysphasia).

Tips
- Ask whether you could examine the patient for signs of (right) hemiplegia.
- Receptive aphasia could be an isolated finding, and the patient may be mislabelled as confused.
- Many patients have a combination of both types of aphasia (global aphasia).
- Naming is impaired in all forms of aphasia, and is therefore not usually of any localisation value.
- An isolation impairment in repetition is called *conductive aphasia*, and is usually due to a lesion in the arcuate fasciculus.

Discussion
Q: Where is the lesion?
- (a) Receptive aphasia: in the superior temporal gyrus in the dominant (left) hemisphere.
- (b) Expressive aphasia: in the inferior frontal gyrus in the dominant (left) hemisphere.

Q: What is the cause of the aphasia?
- Stroke.
- Brain tumours.

Q: How would you investigate?
- Brain CT/MRI.
- Carotid ultrasound examination.
- Assessment of risk factors for stroke.

Q: What is the treatment?
- Treat the underlying cause.

PITFALLS

Pitfalls

- Testing of the first cranial nerve, the gag reflex and the sensation of the tongue is not usually required in exams.
- Slight blurring of the nasal margin of the optic disc is not papilloedema.
- Slight pallor of the temporal part of the optic disc is not optic atrophy.
- Absent venous pulsation with normal-looking optic disc margins could be seen in around 25% of the general population.
- Normal rhythmic variation in the size of the pupil when exposed to light is not a relative afferent pupillary defect (the pupil keeps constricting and slightly dilating several times per second when exposed to light). This is a normal phenomenon called hippus.
- Diplopia could be present even in the absence of abnormal eye movements.
- The description of the visual field defect is from the patient's point of view, not that of the examiner.
- Nerve V does not supply the area over the angle of the jaw.
- A minor degree of facial asymmetry without weakness is not a facial palsy.
- Ptosis is not a feature of VIIth nerve palsy.
- You may get a false impression that the tongue is deviating in LMN VIIth nerve palsy.
- Some minor rippling in the tongue is not fasciculation.
- Some jerky movement of the eyes in extreme lateral gaze is not nystagmus.
- Always consider myasthenia gravis when examining patients with ptosis and/or impairment of ocular movement.
- Always remember the differential diagnosis of ptosis, namely IIIrd nerve palsy, Horner's syndrome, myasthenia gravis, myotonic dystrophy and congenital ptosis.
- Rare causes of ptosis include ocular myopathy, mitochondrial disorders and tabes dorsalis.

- Consider aseptic meningitis (due to cancer, lymphoma or sarcoidosis) when there are multiple cranial nerve palsies.
- Argyll Robertson pupils always appear in books, but not in exams or clinical practice! This is supposed to be a small irregular pupil that reacts to accommodation but not to light, due to syphilis (tabes dorsalis).
- Adie's pupil, however, is occasionally seen in neurology clinics. It is a unilateral dilated pupil that does not react to light (or shows only a sluggish reaction) in young or middle-aged women. Holmes–Adie syndrome is a combination of Adie's pupil and reduced or absent tendon reflexes.
- Rinne's test: hold a 256 or 512 Hz tuning fork in front of the external auditory meatus and then against the mastoid. In the affected ear, air conduction is less than bone conduction in conductive deafness, and air conduction is greater than bone conduction in sensorineural deafness.
- Weber's test: place a 256 or 512 Hz tuning fork in the middle of the forehead. The sound will be louder in the affected ear in conductive deafness, and will be louder in the normal ear in sensorineural deafness.

SECTION II

Examination of the upper limbs

INSTRUCTION A

Examine the upper limbs

Instruction A: Examine the upper limbs
What should you do?

First do the essential. This should include the following:

Inspection

- Ask the patient to place their upper limbs outstretched in front of them with their eyes closed and palms facing upward (pronator test). This will give you a quick indication of any problems with power (drifting down), position sense (fingers move up and down – pseudo-athetosis) or cerebellar disease (arms move up).
- Muscle wasting.
- Muscle fasciculation.
- Scars could be relevant (burn marks may suggest syringomyelia).
- Examine the patients's back for spinal scar or scapular winging.

Tone

- Ensure that the patient is not in pain.
- Ensure that the patient is relaxed.
- Move each upper limb passively. Feel the tone mainly at the elbow and the wrist by flexing and extending the joints.
- Feel for the 'supinator catch' at the wrist by supination and pronation of the forearm.

Power

- Check shoulder abduction (deltoid, C5) by asking the patient to form a wing and then resist you pushing down on their shoulders.
- Check elbow flexion (biceps, C5/6) by asking the patient to pull the *supinated* forearm against your hand. Then ask the patient to pull the forearm *(midway between pronation and supination)* against your hand (brachioradialis, C5/C6).
- Check elbow extension (triceps, C7) by asking the patient to push their forearm against your hand.

- Check finger extension (extensor digitorum, C7) by asking the patient to keep their fingers straight and resist you pressing them down.
- Check the first dorsal interosseous muscle (T1) by asking the patient to push their index finger against your finger.
- Check the abductor pollicis brevis (T1) by asking the patient to move their thumb toward the ceiling against your thumb.

Reflexes
- Use the full length of the tendon hammer and let it swing fully.
- Check biceps (C5), supinator (C6) and triceps (C7) reflexes. Look for muscle contraction, not just the jerky movement.

Coordination
- Demonstrate to the patient how to perform the finger–nose test by taking the patients's finger, pointing to their nose and then to your finger tip.
- Now ask the patient to do this.

Sensory examination
- Always teach the patient first by starting at the sternum or the forehead. The patient needs to recognise normal sensation!
- Test the pain sensation by using the sharp end of a Neurotip.
- Start from the hand and work up. Test random points covering the outer and inner aspects of the hands, the forearms and the arms. This should cover all dermatomes.
- Assess the joint position sense. Hold the distal interphalangeal joint of the middle finger between your two fingers from the sides and move it up and down. Make only a small movement (2–3 mm), and avoid putting the joint in extreme positions. First show the patient what you are going to do, and then ask them to do it with their eyes closed.
- Test for vibration sense. Start with the wrist, and if that is abnormal, move to the elbow and shoulder.

At the end
Ask whether you could examine the lower limbs.

Tips

- Take time to explain each step of the examination to the patient (e.g. finger–nose test). This will save time and ensure the correct technique.
- It is important to use the Medical Research Council scale when describing muscle weakness (grade 0, no *visible* contraction; grade 1, flicker of contraction; grade 2, movement with gravity; grade 3, movement against gravity; grade 4, movement against partial resistance; grade 5, normal power).
- Grade the power according to the maximum power achieved.
- When examining muscle power, test each side and then compare them.
- Examination of muscles such as the serratus anterior, rhomboids, supraspinatus and infraspinatus is rarely needed in the exam setting.
- When reflexes are absent, do the reinforcement by asking the patient to clench their teeth.
- Grade the reflexes as absent, normal or brisk.
- Remember that asymmetry of reflexes is usually significant.
- Sensory examination should be performed at the end of the examination of the upper limbs. By that stage you should have some idea about the possible diagnosis. The sensory findings should complement the motor ones. When you examine pinprick sensation, ask the patient 'Does the pin feel sharp as it did on your chest or forehead?' Do *not* ask 'Can you feel it?', as the answer will be yes!
- There is no need to ask the patient to close their eyes during the pinprick examination, as it would serve no purpose. However, some general physicians still insist that the patient closes their eyes, so you may have to do it!

- Light touch examination does not usually add anything to the findings, so do it at the end, if you still have time.
- Test the vibration sense with a 128 Hz tuning fork.
- Always think as you are examining the patient. It is a good idea to have a summary of the findings in your head before reporting to the examiner.

FINDINGS

Finding One

There is right/left arm weakness with increased tone and brisk reflexes. Also there is (possible) impairment of pinprick sensation over the right/left arm.

Diagnosis
- Right/left monoplegia (could be part of right/left hemiplegia).

Tips
- Ask whether you could examine the lower limbs.
- In a case of hemiplegia, the patient could have a hemiplegic gait. In this case the lower limb moves in a semicircle, the toe scraping the floor with each step, and the arm is held in a flexed position close to the chest.
- Look at the face to see whether there is evidence of facial weakness (ipsilateral UMN lesion of nerve VII).
- Ask whether you could assess the visual field and the speech.

Discussion
Q: What are the causes of monoplegia (or hemiplegia)?
- Cerebrovascular disease (sudden onset).
- Brain tumour (gradual onset).
- Cervical cord lesion (gradual onset).

Q: How would you investigate?
- Brain CT and/or MRI.
- MRI of cervical spine.
- Assessment of vascular risk factors such as blood sugar and cholesterol levels.

Q: What is the treatment?
- Treat the underlying cause.
- Treat the vascular risk factors.

Finding Two

There is generalised wasting and weakness (possibly fasciculation) of the small muscles of both hands, with dorsal guttering. The reflexes are brisk (or may be absent). There are no sensory signs.

Diagnosis
- Motor neurone disease.

Tips
- Ask whether you could look at the tongue.
- Ask whether you could look at the trunk and the lower limbs for fasciculation.

Discussion
Q: What is the differential diagnosis?
- Cervical spondylotic myelopathy (there are usually sensory signs).
- Syringomyelia (dissociated sensory loss, scars from burns, absent reflexes).
- Combined ulnar and median nerve lesions.
- Charcot–Marie–Tooth disease.
- Disuse atrophy, as for example in rheumatological diseases.

Q: What are the causes of wasting in only one hand?
- Any of the above.
- Thoracic outlet syndrome.
- Pancoast's tumour.
- Brachial plexus lesion, such as trauma or malignant infiltration.

Q: How would you investigate?
- NCS/EMG: important to confirm the diagnosis.
- MRI of the cervical spine.

Q: What is the treatment?
- Multi-disciplinary care.
- Riluzole.
- Gastrostomy and non-invasive ventilation.
- Palliative care.

Finding Three

There is generalised wasting and weakness of the small muscles of the right/left hand, which are more prominent in the first dorsal interosseous muscle, but sparing of the thenar eminence. There is impairment of pinprick sensation over the little finger, the medial half of the ring finger and the medial side of the hand (to the level of the wrist). There may also be a claw hand (hyperextension at the metacarpophalangeal joints and flexion at the interphalangeal joints of the little and ring fingers).

Diagnosis
- Ulnar nerve entrapment at the elbow.

Tips
- If the sensory signs extend to the elbow, the lesion is at C8/T1 level.
- Look for any evidence of scars around the elbow.

Discussion
Q: What are the causes of ulnar nerve entrapment at the elbow?
- Chronic compression due to old fracture, or dislocation at the elbow or osteoarthritic change.
- Acute compression of the ulnar nerve after a general anaesthesia.
- Occupational causes (e.g. the condition occurring in a painter, bricklayer or secretary).
- Part of mononeuritis multiplex.
- Other causes of wasting of the small muscle of the hands (*see* page 68) could resemble ulnar nerve palsy.

Q: How would you investigate?
- NCS/EMG: important to confirm the diagnosis and determine the level of the lesion.

Q: What is the treatment?

- Usually conservative treatment and, if possible, avoidance of further compression.
- Ulnar nerve decompression or transposition could be considered in severe cases.

Finding Four

There is wasting of the thenar eminence and weakness of the abductor pollicis brevis of the right/left hand. There is also sensory loss over the palmar aspects of the thumb, index and middle fingers and the lateral half of the ring finger.

Diagnosis
- Right/left median nerve palsy (likely to be carpal tunnel syndrome).

Tips
- Carpal tunnel syndrome is five times more common in women than in men, as women have a narrower cross-sectional area in the carpal tunnel than do men.
- Look for previous surgical scars.
- The patient may also have weakness in flexion and opposition of the thumb.
- Test the flexor pollicis longus (by flexing the distal phalanx of the thumb) and the flexor digitorum profundus I and II (by flexing the distal phalanx of the index finger). If they are intact, the lesion is below the origin of the anterior interosseous nerve, confirming the diagnosis of carpal tunnel syndrome.
- Check Tinel's sign with percussion over the palmar side of the wrist to produce paraesthesia over the median nerve distribution.

Discussion
Q: What are the causes of carpal tunnel syndrome?
- Idiopathic (common in neurology clinics!).
- Endocrine disorders such as hypothyroidism, diabetes and acromegaly.
- Rheumatological diseases such as rheumatoid arthritis and osteoarthritis.
- Other causes, such as pregnancy, the oral contraceptive pill, and amyloidosis.

Q: What are the characteristic sensory symptoms of carpal tunnel syndrome?
- Painful paraesthesia in the hand and fingers, which may radiate up to the level of the elbow.
- Symptoms worse at night.
- Symptoms relieved by shaking of the hands.

Q: How would you investigate?
- Thyroid function test and blood glucose levels.
- Upper limbs NCS.

Q: What is the treatment?
- Diuretics.
- Wrist splint.
- Local steroid injection.
- Surgical decompression.

Finding Five

There is weakness in dorsiflexion of the wrist (wrist drop) and the patient is unable to straighten the fingers due to weakness of the finger extensors at the metacarpophalangeal joints.

Diagnosis
- Right/left radial nerve palsy.

Tips
- If the patient's wrist is passively extended, they will be able to straighten the fingers at the interphalangeal joints but not at the metacarpophalangeal joints as the interossei and lumbricals are functioning normally.
- The extensor digitorum, extensor indicis and extensor carpi ulnaris are the main wrist extensors, all of which are supplied by the radial nerve.
- Abduction and adduction of the fingers may appear weak unless they are tested when the wrist is rested flat.
- Due to overlap in the sensory supply by the median, ulnar and radial nerves, only a small area of impairment sensation in the skin over the first dorsal interosseous muscle could be affected in radial nerve palsy.
- Always test the triceps and the brachioradialis, as they may be affected if the lesion of the radial nerve is high (above the middle third of the humerus).

Discussion
Q: What are the causes of radial nerve palsy?
- Acute compression at the 'spiral groove' after a general anaesthetic or being unconscious (Saturday night palsy!).
- Fractured shaft of the humerus.
- Crutch trauma at the level of the axilla (rare).

Q: What is Saturday night palsy?
- Acute compression of the radial nerve as it passes down the posterior aspect of the humerus in the spiral groove. This tends to occur in people who are drunk and who fall asleep with the arm hanging over the side of an armchair. The triceps is spared.

Q: How would you investigate?
- Upper limbs NCS.

Q: What is the treatment?
- Wrist splint.
- Physiotherapy.

Q: What is the prognosis?
- Full recovery usually occurs in cases of acute compression. The outcome after humerus fracture is variable.

PITFALLS

Pitfalls

- You could find signs of ataxia when you are asked to examine the upper limbs. If that is the case, you have to demonstrate all of the other features of ataxia (*see* page 111).
- You could find signs of parkinsonism when you are asked to examine the upper limbs. If that is the case, you have to demonstrate all of the other features of parkinsonism (*see* page 113).
- It is unlikely that you will be asked to see a patient with chorea (characterised by brief, abrupt and fidgety involuntary movements which flit randomly around the body). The most common cause of chorea in neurology clinics is dyskinesia due to levodopa in patients with Parkinson's disease. Other causes include Huntington's disease, Sydenham's chorea, systemic lupus erythematosus, oral contraceptive pill, thyrotoxicosis, polycythaemia and neuro-acanthocytosis. Neuroleptics could also cause tardive dyskinesia, such as orofacial dyskinesia, including lip-smacking, chewing and grimacing.
- As you are doing the examination, always think whether the lesion is central (brain and spinal cord) or peripheral (nerves, muscles and neuromuscular junction). UMN signs (increased tone and brisk reflexes) are usually an indication of a central lesion. LMN signs (reduced tone, wasting, fasciculation and absent reflexes) are usually an indication of a peripheral lesion.
- Pyramidal weakness (UMN) predominantly affects shoulder abduction, elbow extension and finger extension (the extensors).
- Inverted supinator tendon reflex (diminished or absent supinator reflex with reflex contraction of finger flexors) indicates cord and root lesion at C5 level.
- The radial nerve supplies all extensors of the arm. The ulnar nerve supplies all intrinsic muscles of the hand *except* the

lateral two lumbricals, opponens pollicis, abductor pollicis brevis and flexor pollicis brevis (LOAF), which are supplied by the median nerve.

- Remember that all of the intrinsic muscles of the hand are supplied by T1.
- If there is dermatomal impairment of pinprick sensation, map the abnormality (e.g. C8/T1). Start from the abnormal area and move to the normal area.
- There are four patterns of sensory loss. Glove (or stocking in the lower limbs) distribution indicates peripheral neuropathy, sensory level indicates spinal cord lesion, hemianaesthesia indicates a contralateral cerebral lesion, and dissociated sensory loss (impaired spinothalamic and preserved posterior column) indicates Brown–Séquard syndrome or anterior spinal artery syndrome.

SECTION III

Examination of the lower limbs and gait

INSTRUCTION A

Examine the lower limbs

Instruction A: Examine the lower limbs
What should you do?

First do the essential. This should include the following:

Inspection

- Muscle wasting.
- Muscle fasciculation.
- Any deformities, such as pes cavus or asymmetry of the leg length (one leg shorter than the other).
- Any scar (usually not relevant!).
- Examine the patients's back for spinal scars.

Tone

- Check whether the patient is in pain.
- Feel the tone at the knee by passively and rapidly flexing and extending the knee.
- Check the tone at the ankle by flexing and dorsiflexing the foot.
- Check the ankle clonus at the same time by holding the knee in a semi-flexed position and pushing the foot up suddenly with moderate force.

Power

- Check the hip flexion (L1/2) by asking the patient to push their thigh against your hand with the knee flexed at 90 degrees.
- Check the knee flexion (L5/S1) by asking the patient to bend their knee against your hand. Then ask them to push the knee out against your hand to test knee extension (L3/4).
- Check the ankle dorsiflexion (L4/L5) by asking the patient to push up their foot against your hand. Also check the ankle plantar flexion (S1) by asking the patient to push their foot down against your hand.

Reflexes
- Use the full length of the tendon hammer, and let it swing fully.
- Check knee (L3/4) and ankle (S1/2) reflexes. Look for the muscle contraction, not just the jerky movement.
- Test the plantar response. Use the orange stick, not the sharp end of the tendon hammer. Start with the outer part of the sole and move towards the base of the big toe.

Coordination
- Demonstrate to the patient how to do the heel–shin test by taking the heel of the patient, putting it just below the knee and running it down the shin and taking it up again below the knee.
- Now ask the patient to do this.

Sensory examination
- Always teach the patient to recognise normal sensation first by starting at the sternum or the forehead. The patient needs to know the normal sensation!
- Test the pain sensation by using the sharp end of a Neurotip.
- Start from the feet and move upward. Do random points covering the outer and inner aspects of the feet, the calves and the thighs. This should cover all dermatomes.
- Test the joint position sense. Hold the big toe at the sides and move it up and down. Make only small movements (2–3 mm), and avoid putting the joint in an extreme position. First show the patient what you are going to do, and then do it with the patient's eyes closed.
- Test for vibration sense. Start with the ankle (medial malleolus), and if this is abnormal move to the knee and iliac crest.

At the end
Ask whether you could examine the gait and the upper limbs.

Tips

- Be thorough when explaining to the patient each step of the examination (e.g. heel–shin test). This will save time and ensure that the correct technique is used.
- Remember to use the Medical Research Council scale when describing muscle weakness (*see* page 63).
- There is no need to perform hip extension, adduction or abduction, foot inversion or eversion and extension of the big toe, unless this is clinically indicated (e.g. in cases of foot drop).
- If reflexes are absent, do the reinforcement by asking the patient to hold the fingers of both hands together and pull them against each other.
- Grade the reflexes as absent, normal or brisk.
- Ankle reflex could be elicited by the plantar strike technique. Place your fingers on the sole of the patient's foot, which should be in passive dorsiflexed position, and strike your fingers.
- When you examine pinprick sensation, ask the patient 'Does the pin feel sharp as it did on your chest or forehead?' Do *not* ask 'Can you feel it?', as the answer will be yes!
- There is no need to ask the patient to close their eyes during the pinprick examination, as it would serve no purpose. However, some general physicians still insist that the patient closes their eyes, so you may have to do it!
- If there is dermatomal impairment of pinprick sensation, map the abnormality (e.g. L5/S1).
- Test the vibration sense with a 128 Hz tuning fork.
- Light touch examination does not usually add anything to the findings, so do it at the end, if you still have time.
- Always think as you are examining the patient. It is a good idea to have a summary of the findings in your head before reporting to the examiner.

FINDINGS

Finding One

Bilateral increased (spastic) tone with brisk reflexes, and upgoing plantars. There is (possible) weakness, ankle clonus, sensory level or disuse wasting.

Diagnosis
- Spastic paraparesis.

Tips
- Examination of the gait will show a stiff, scissor gait with the legs crossing in front of each other while the patient is walking.
- Check for any sensory level.
- Ask whether you could examine the upper limbs. At least test the reflexes, as this will help to localise the lesion.
- Multiple sclerosis is a common cause of spastic paraparesis in young patients. Again ask if you could examine the upper limbs, elicit cerebellar signs and look at the optic discs.
- Examine the back for any scars.

Discussion
Q: What are the main causes of spastic paraparesis?
- Multiple sclerosis in young patients.
- Cervical spondylotic myelopathy in middle-aged and elderly patients.
- Spinal trauma.
- Spinal tumours (primary or metastatic).
- Vascular causes, such as spinal arteriovenous malformation and spinal ischaemia (anterior spinal artery syndrome).

Q: What are the other causes of spastic paraparesis?
- Vitamin B_{12} deficiency.
- Thoracic cord meningioma in middle-aged women.
- Motor neurone disease.
- Hereditary spastic paraplegia.

- Tropical spastic paraplegia.
- Parasagittal meningioma.
- Radiation myelopathy.
- Syringomyelia.

Q: How would you investigate?
- MRI of brain.
- MRI of spine.
- Cerebrospinal fluid analysis looking in particular for oligoclonal bands.
- Other investigations if there is a clear indication as to the cause (e.g. NCS/EMG in motor neurone disease, checking vitamin B_{12} levels).

Q: What is the treatment?
- Treat the underlying cause, which may involve surgery in patients with cervical spondylotic myelopathy.

Finding Two

There is a reduction in pinprick sensation in the stocking distribution. There is also impairment of vibration and joint position sense. Ankle jerks may be absent.

Diagnosis
- Predominantly sensory peripheral neuropathy.

Tips
- Ask whether you could examine the upper limb to demonstrate impairment of sensation in the glove distribution.

Discussion
Q: What are the causes of predominantly sensory peripheral neuropathy?
- Diabetes.
- Vitamin B deficiency (thiamine and vitamin B_{12}), especially in alcoholics.
- Paraneoplastic neuropathy.
- Drugs such as anti-tuberculosis (isoniazid and ethambutol) and chemotherapeutic agents (cyclosporin, cisplatin and vincristine).
- Others causes, such as amyloidosis and chronic renal failure.
- Idiopathic, especially in elderly patients.
- Paraproteinaemic neuropathy (mixed sensory and motor neuropathy).

Q: How would you investigate?
- NCS/EMG: important to confirm the diagnosis.
- Blood sugar levels.
- Full blood count and ESR.
- Liver function test.
- Vitamin B_{12} levels.

- Vasculitic screen.
- Paraprotein screen.
- Other investigations, such as paraneoplastic antibodies and sural nerve biopsy, may be needed in some patients.

Q: What is the treatment?
- Treat the underlying cause if possible.
- Symptomatic treatment with tricyclic antidepressants, carbamazepine or gabapentin.

Finding Three

Bilateral generalised weakness that is more marked distally, with absent jerks and mild impairment of pinprick, joint position and vibration sense.

Diagnosis

- Predominantly motor peripheral neuropathy (likely to be Guillain–Barré syndrome).

Tips

- Ask whether you could examine the upper limbs.
- Look for any evidence of bilateral facial weakness (LMN lesion of nerve VII) and any bulbar involvement.
- Ask whether there has been an antecedent upper respiratory tract infection or diarrhoea.

Discussion

Q: What are the causes of predominantly motor peripheral neuropathy?

- Guillain–Barré syndrome.
- Chronic inflammatory demyelinating polyradiculoneuropathy (CIDP).
- Charcot–Marie–Tooth disease.
- Porphyria.
- Lead poisoning.

Q: How would you investigate?

- NCS/EMG: important to confirm the diagnosis and determine whether there is any axonal neuropathy (Guillain–Barré syndrome is usually a demyelinating neuropathy).
- Cerebrospinal fluid analysis, looking in particular for high protein levels.
- Vitamin B_{12} levels.
- Vasculitic screen.
- Paraprotein screen.

- Serum ganglioside antibodies.
- Porphyria screen.

Q: What is the treatment of Guillain–Barré syndrome?
- Regular monitoring of forced vital capacity, as the patient is at risk of respiratory failure.
- Regular monitoring of blood pressure and heart rhythm, as the patient is at risk of autonomic neuropathy.
- Low-dose subcutaneous heparin to prevent venous thrombo-embolism.
- Intensive-care support, as ventilation may be needed.
- Intravenous immunoglobulin.
- Neurorehabilitation.

Q: What is the prognosis of Guillain–Barré syndrome?
- Around 80% of patients make a complete recovery after 1 year. About 5% die and 15% are still unable to walk unaided after 1 year.

Finding Four

There is right/left leg weakness with increased tone and brisk reflexes. Right/left upgoing plantars. There may also be impairment of pinprick sensation over the right/left leg.

Diagnosis

- Right/left monoplegia (likely to be part of right/left hemiplegia).

Tips

- Ask whether you could examine the upper limbs.
- In the case of hemiplegia, the patient could have a hemiplegic gait (*see* page 67).
- Examine the face to see whether there is evidence of facial weakness (ipsilateral UMN lesion of nerve VII).
- Ask whether you could assess the visual field and the speech.
- If there is loss of joint position and vibration on the monoparetic side, and loss of pain and temperature on the opposite side to a certain sensory level (e.g. T10), the diagnosis is Brown–Séquard syndrome.

Discussion

Q: What are the causes of monoplegia?
- Cerebrovascular disease (sudden onset).
- Brain tumour (gradual onset).
- Spinal cord lesion (gradual onset).

Q: What are the causes of hemiplegia?
- Cerebrovascular disease (sudden onset).
- Brain tumour (gradual onset).
- Cervical cord lesion (gradual onset).

Q: What are the causes of Brown–Séquard syndrome?
- Spinal cord tumour.
- Multiple sclerosis.

Q: How would you investigate?
- CT and/or MRI of brain.
- MRI of spine.
- Assessment of vascular risk factors, such as blood sugar and cholesterol levels.

Q: What is the treatment?
- Treat the underlying cause.
- Treat the vascular risk factors.

Finding Five

Bilateral distal wasting and weakness of ankle dorsiflexion (bilateral foot drop). Absent ankle and knee jerks. Pes cavus.

Diagnosis
- Charcot–Marie–Tooth disease (CMT).

Tips
- CMT is also known as hereditary motor and sensory neuropathy.
- CMT causes predominantly motor peripheral neuropathy.
- Ask whether you could examine the upper limbs, as there may be wasting of the small muscles of the hand and absent reflexes.
- The degree of disability is usually minimal, despite the marked neurological signs.
- The patient could have a high steppage gait (*see* page 101).

Discussion
Q: What is the mode of inheritance?
- Mainly autosomal dominant. Recessive and X-linked modes of inheritance have also been reported.

Q: What are the different types of CMT?
- CMT1: demyelinating neuropathy.
- CMT2: axonal neuropathy.

Q: How would you investigate?
- NCS/EMG.
- Genetic testing, duplication of the gene PMP-22 (peripheral myelin protein-22).

Q: What is the treatment?
- Genetic counselling.
- Supportive measures such as physiotherapy and splints.

Finding Six

There is weakness in dorsiflexion of the right/left ankle and eversion of the right/left foot. There is a (possible) reduction in pinprick sensation over the lateral aspect of the calf and the dorsum of the foot. Ankle jerk is preserved.

Diagnosis
- Right/left foot drop due to common peroneal nerve palsy.

Tips
- Examine the dorsiflexion of the big toe by asking the patient to move the toe against resistance (extensor hallucis longus).
- Inversion of the foot is normal in common peroneal nerve palsy.
- The common peroneal nerve has two branches, namely the superficial and deep branches. If the lesion is below the origin of the superficial branch, the sensory changes will be confined to a small zone in the dorsal area between the big toe and the second toe.
- The patient could have a steppage gait, as seen by lifting the foot high during walking to avoid scraping the toes and foot slapping.

Discussion
Q: What are the causes of foot drop?
- Injury to the common peroneal nerve, usually at the level of the fibula, as a result of trauma or compression.
- L5 root lesion if the inversion of the ankle is also weak. L5 root lesion is usually painful.
- Sciatic nerve lesion if there is weakness of the toe, plantar flexion and loss of ankle jerk (involvement of the tibial nerve).
- It could be part of a generalised neurological problem, such as peripheral neuropathy, motor neurone disease (ankle reflex will be brisk with no sensory signs) or cauda equina lesion.

Q: How would you investigate?
- NCS/EMG.

Q: What is the treatment?
- Treat the underlying cause if possible.
- Ankle splint.

Finding Seven

There is weakness mainly in hip flexion and extension. The patient has difficulty in standing from a sitting position.

Diagnosis
- Proximal myopathy.

Tips
- Ask whether you could examine the upper limbs for signs of proximal myopathy.
- Ask whether you could examine the gait (waddling gait; *see* page 115).

Discussion
Q: What are the causes of proximal myopathy?
- Polymyositis or dermatomyositis.
- Inclusion body myositis, which is the most common form of myopathy after the age of 50 years.
- Endocrine causes: Cushing's syndrome and thyrotoxicosis.
- Drugs: steroids, amiodarone, lithium and statins.
- Alcoholism.
- Limb girdle dystrophy.
- Metabolic myopathies.
- Osteomalacia.
- Paraneoplastic myopathy (very rare).

Q: How would you investigate?
- Investigations will depend on the possible cause.
- Blood tests, such as thyroid function test.
- Muscle enzymes.
- EMG.
- Muscle biopsy.
- Genetic testing.

Q: What is the treatment?

- Treat the underlying cause. Give medication such as corticosteroids and azathioprine in cases of polymyositis and dermatomyositis.

INSTRUCTION B

Examine the gait

Instruction B: Examine the gait
What should you do?

- You will probably be asked to examine the relevant part of the nervous system as you see fit following the gait examination. However, you may be asked to specifically examine part of the nervous system, such as the lower limbs, after the gait examination.
- Have a very quick look all around. Young patients are more likely to have an ataxic or waddling gait, whereas elderly patients probably have Parkinson's disease or stroke.
- Examine the face for any evidence of parkinsonism.
- Look for any evidence of resting or action tremor.
- Look very carefully at the gait base (wide or narrow), the steps, the arms (whether or not they swing), posture (whether or not it is stooped) and the ability to turn.
- Ask the patient to do the tandem walk (heel-to-toe). Demonstrate this to the patient first.
- Stand close to the patient to prevent them from falling during the exam!

Tips

- If you think the patient is ataxic, perform Romberg's test. Ask the patient to stand with their feet together and their arms by their sides. Then ask them to close their eyes.
- Romberg's sign tends to be overrated. All patients with ataxia tend to get worse when they close their eyes. Romberg's sign should only be considered positive if there is a significant degree of worsening of the ataxia after closing the eyes, which indicates sensory ataxia.

FINDINGS

Finding One

The patient's gait is wide-based with difficulty performing the heel-to-toe test ('drunken gait').

Diagnosis
- Ataxic gait due to cerebellar syndrome.

Tips
- Check the cerebellar signs, namely nystagmus, dysarthria, abnormal finger–nose test and abnormal heel–shin test.
- Look for intention tremor (worse on approaching the target).
- Test for dysdiadochokinesia, which is defined as a breakdown of rhythmic, rapid alternating movements (impairment of rapid pronation and supination movements of one hand on the other one).
- Look for any evidence of increased tone, spastic legs or optic atrophy (indicative of multiple sclerosis). Look for any signs of alcoholic liver disease.

Discussion
Q: What are the causes of cerebellar syndrome?
- Multiple sclerosis.
- Alcoholic cerebellar degeneration (usually gait ataxia).
- Drugs such as anticonvulsants (phenytoin and carbamazepine) and lithium.
- Stroke-related causes, such as ischaemia or haemorrhage.
- Paraneoplastic syndrome (usually with lung and breast cancer).
- Spinocerebellar ataxia (genetic ataxia).
- Idiopathic cerebellar ataxia.
- Friedreich's ataxia (pes cavus, absent ankle jerks, upgoing plantars, and scoliosis).
- Posterior fossa tumours.
- Hypothyroidism.

Q: How would you investigate?
- Investigations are based on the likely cause.
- MRI of brain.
- Cerebrospinal fluid analysis, looking in particular for oligoclonal bands.
- Anticonvulsant levels in the blood.
- Paraneoplastic antibodies.
- Genetic testing for spinocerebellar ataxia.
- Chest X-ray or mammogram.
- NCS/EMG and genetic testing for Friedreich's ataxia (DNA testing for GAA repeats of the frataxin gene).

Q: What is the treatment?
- Treat the underlying cause if possible.
- Genetic counselling.

Finding Two

Patient walks with small steps and shuffles. They stoop, with lack of arm swing. The arms are held in flexed positions.

Diagnosis
- Parkinson's disease.

Tips
- Look for pill-rolling tremor.
- Examine the face. It is usually expressionless with lack of blinking.
- Examine for rigidity (cog-wheel if there is tremor), by slow flexion and extension movements at the wrist. If rigidity is mild, ask the patient to flex and extend their fingers in the contralateral hand to reinforce the rigidity.
- Demonstrate bradykinesia by asking the patient to repetitively open and close their thumb and index finger. Observe both the slowness and reduction of the amplitude of the movement.
- Symptoms and signs of Parkinson's disease are more prominent on one side (asymmetry).

Discussion
Q: What is the differential diagnosis of the parkinsonian syndrome?
- Drug-induced parkinsonism, mainly caused by phenothiazines.
- Vascular parkinsonism (multiple cerebral infarct state).
- Progressive supranuclear palsy (check for vertical gaze palsy).
- Multiple system atrophy (check the blood pressure with the patient lying and standing).

Q: How do you make the diagnosis of Parkinson's disease?
- It is a clinical diagnosis.

Q: What is the treatment?
- Drugs are the main form of treatment.
- Dopamine agonists, especially in the early stages of the disease and in young patients (ropinirole, pramipexole and rotigotine).
- Levodopa is still the main and most effective treatment.
- Monoamine oxidase B inhibitors (rasagiline and selegiline).
- Catechol-O-methyl transferase (COMT) inhibitors (entacapone).
- Apomorphine injection and infusion.
- Surgery, mainly deep brain stimulation. Patient selection is crucial. Patients should have positive responsiveness to dopamine therapy with no cognitive or psychiatric problems.

Q: What are the main problems with levodopa therapy?
- Wearing off: the response period becomes shorter and shorter.
- Dyskinesia: excessive involuntary choreiform movements.
- On/off: rapid and unpredictable shift from 'on' state (good response) to 'off' state (lack of response).

Finding Three

Patients's legs held wide apart. Lumbar lordosis. Trunk moving from side to side with pelvis dropping.

Diagnosis

- Waddling gait due to hereditary muscular dystrophies (Becker muscular dystrophy).

Tips

- A male patient.
- You are unlikely to see Duchenne muscular dystrophy, as patients are usually severely disabled if they reach adulthood.
- Look for pseudohypertrophy of the calves.
- The upper limbs may be involved in the later stages.
- The facial muscles are usually intact.

Discussion

Q: What is the mode of inheritance of Becker muscular dystrophy?

- X-linked (there is not always a family history, as 30% of the cases are new mutations).

Q: What are the other causes of waddling gait?

- Any cause of proximal myopathy (*see* page 103).

Q: How would you investigate?

- Serum creatinine kinase.
- EMG.
- Muscle biopsy.

Q: What is the treatment?

- There is no specific treatment, and therapy is mainly supportive.
- Respiratory and cardiac monitoring.
- Genetic counselling.

PITFALLS

Pitfalls

- Remember that asymmetry of reflexes should be regarded as abnormal.
- When the big toe moves up in the upgoing plantar response (UMN sign), the other four toes fan and turn towards the sole.
- Pyramidal weakness (UMN) predominantly affects hip flexor, knee flexors and ankle dorsiflexion (the flexors).
- Absent ankle reflexes and reduced vibration sense in an elderly patient could be normal.
- Sensory examination should be performed at the end of the examination of the lower limbs. By that stage you should have some idea about the possible diagnosis. The sensory findings should complement the motor ones (e.g. reduced pinprick sensation in stocking distribution in patients with absent ankle jerks).
- Your sensory examination should aim to demonstrate a sensory level (in spastic paraparesis), stocking distribution of sensory impairment (in peripheral neuropathy) and dermatomal abnormalities (L5/S1 in drop foot).
- As you are doing the examination, always think whether the lesion is central (brain and spinal cord) or peripheral (nerves, muscles and neuromuscular junction). UMN signs (increased tone, brisk reflexes and upgoing plantars) are usually an indication of a central lesion. LMN signs (reduced tone, fasciculation, absent reflexes, downgoing or absent plantar response) are usually an indication of a peripheral lesion.
- Patients with sensory ataxia usually have severe impairment of joint position and vibration with positive Romberg's sign. Such patients usually stamp their feet on the floor when walking. Sensory ataxia is usually due to subacute combined degeneration of the cord (vitamin B_{12} deficiency) and tabes dorsalis (very rare).

- Any cause of severe sensory neuropathy could lead to sensory ataxia, such as paraproteinaemic neuropathy and chronic inflammatory demyelinating polyradiculoneuropathy (CIDP).
- Gait apraxia, marche à petits pas and lower body parkinsonism are different terms used to describe patients who walk with short shuffling steps. This is an indication of diffuse cerebrovascular ischaemic disease (small vessel disease).
- The most common cause of absent ankle jerks and extensor plantars in clinical practice is an elderly patient with diabetes and cervical myelopathy. Other causes include subacute combined degeneration of the cord, taboparesis, Friedreich's ataxia, motor neurone disease and conus medullaris lesion.
- The conus is part of the central nervous system (UMN), whereas the cauda equina is part of the peripheral nervous system (LMN). Lesions involve both parts, producing a mixture of UMN and LMN signs.
- Remember that a short leg with LMN signs and no sensory abnormalities indicates old polio.

Index